Adel Aissi

Manual of sutures in veterinary surgery

Adel Aissi

Manual of sutures in veterinary surgery

ScienciaScripts

Imprint

Any brand names and product names mentioned in this book are subject to trademark, brand or patent protection and are trademarks or registered trademarks of their respective holders. The use of brand names, product names, common names, trade names, product descriptions etc. even without a particular marking in this work is in no way to be construed to mean that such names may be regarded as unrestricted in respect of trademark and brand protection legislation and could thus be used by anyone.

Cover image: www.ingimage.com

This book is a translation from the original published under ISBN 978-3-330-87287-5.

Publisher:
Sciencia Scripts
is a trademark of
Dodo Books Indian Ocean Ltd. and OmniScriptum S.R.L publishing group

120 High Road, East Finchley, London, N2 9ED, United Kingdom
Str. Armeneasca 28/1, office 1, Chisinau MD-2012, Republic of Moldova, Europe
Printed at: see last page
ISBN: 978-620-5-84786-2

The ideal suture must meet certain requirements. It must maintain a tensile strength in line with the stresses on the surgical wound. It must be easy to handle and have good knot security. It must be acapillary, non-allergenic and non-carcinogenic.

It must be tissue compatible to minimise local tissue reaction and immune response. It must be able to be reabsorbed once healing is well advanced or be encapsulated without post-operative complications. Environmental conditions, such as the presence of body fluids (serum, urine, pus, etc.) or inflammation, must not excessively affect its rate of resorption. The degradation products must be non-toxic. Finally, this thread must be readily available, at low cost and easily sterilisable. No wire currently meets all of these requirements. It is therefore necessary, for each operation, to look for the wire with the most compatible characteristics for the planned operation. These characteristics differ depending on whether the wire is braided or single-stranded.

THANKS

SLIMANI.C

Who helped me considerably in the execution of this work,

And who surrounds me every day a little more with his love.

I love you.

My son Hydar Nacif

To my parents and sisters,

This work is the culmination of a dream in which you allowed me to believe.

I love you deeply.

To my family-in-law,

For his warm welcome, his simplicity and his kindness.

To all the other members of my family,

whom I did not mention on the paper but whom I do not forget.

TABLE OF CONTENTS:

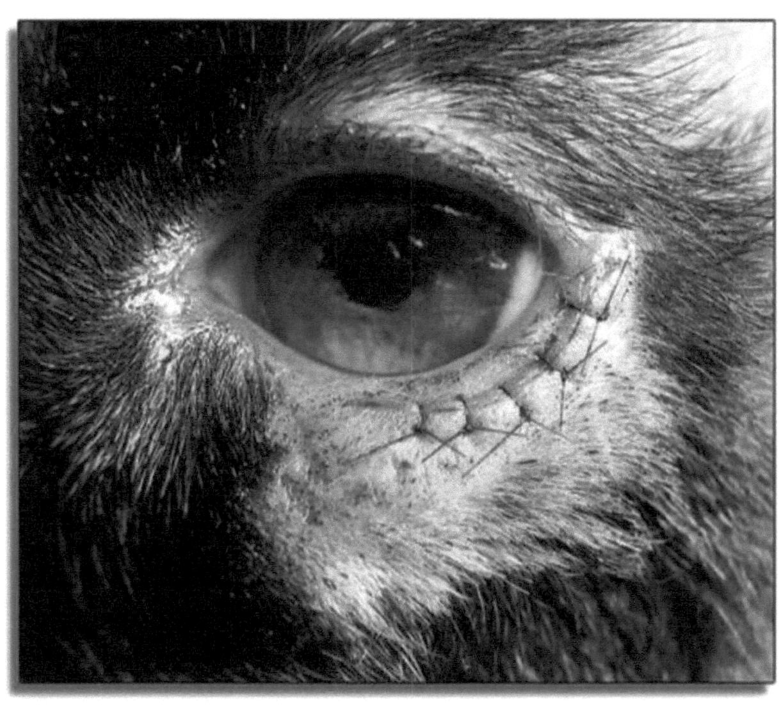

MANUAL OF SUTURES IN VETERINARY SURGERY

By Dr Aissi Adel

CHAPTER 1

<u>Suture materials :</u>

- Lapince.

- The needle gate.

- Sutures.

I / Suture materials :

1- <u>The clamp :</u>

Mouse tooth forceps or various types of trauma forceps are used, depending on the case.

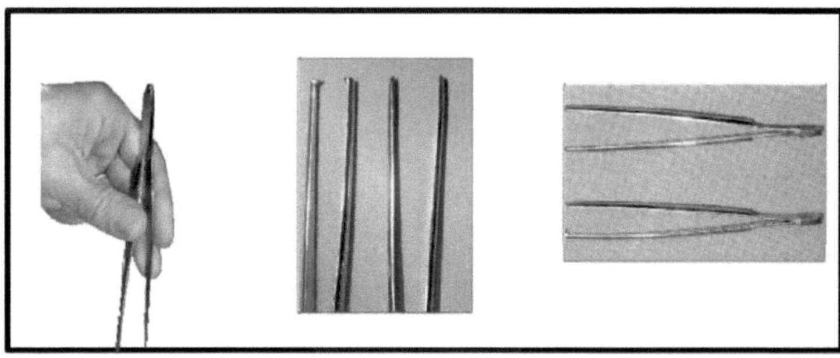

Figure: 01

2- <u>The needle door :</u>

-The curved needles are handled with a needle clamp.

-The needle is gripped near its middle, on the heel side.

-The needle holder is held between the thumb and ring finger on the 2nd or 3rd phalanx.

-The index finger is used to exert the pressure necessary to insert the needle into the wound.

-The needle should always be turned towards the surgeon's thumb.

-Under no circumstances should a needle clamp be used as a haemostatic clamp. The reverse is also true.

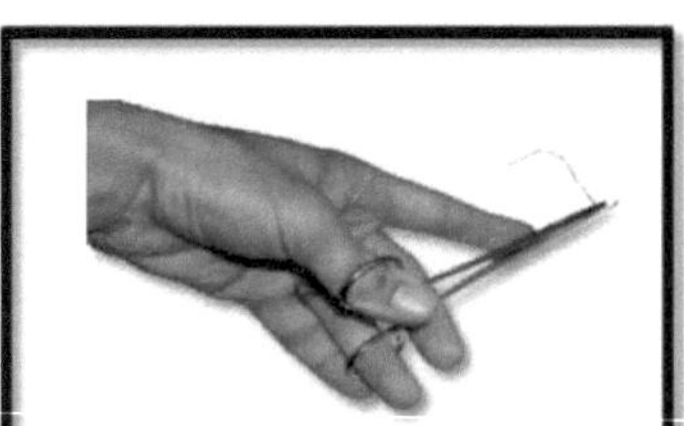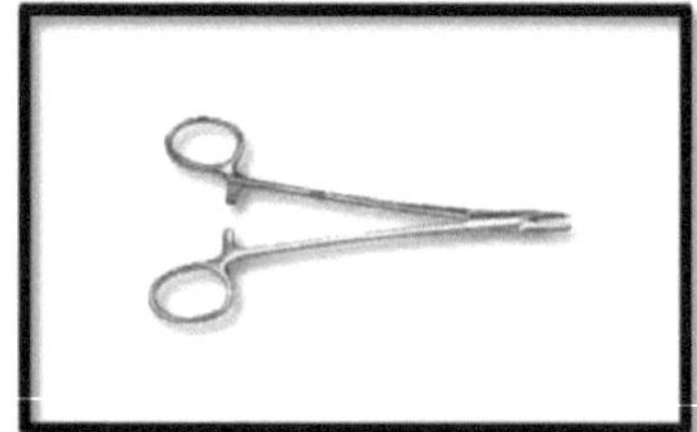

Figure: 02

3- <u>Sutures</u> :

-Sutures are classified according to their tissue behaviour (absorbable or not), their origin (natural or synthetic) and their texture (monobrand or braided).

-In Europe, sutures from animal products (catgut: ruminant mucosa) were phased out in 2001. Silk remains the only natural suture used in veterinary surgery.

Ideally, a non-absorbable suture should retain its strength properties for 60 days.

-Degradation of a suture occurs either by hydrolysis or by phagocytosis. Hydrolysis is a phenomenon without the participation of a cellular contingent, similar to the melting of a sugar cube in water. Phagocytosis involves inflammation cells (mainly macrophages).

3.1 <u>Physical and biological characteristics</u> :

3.1.1 <u>Physical properties</u> :

❖ <u>Wire diameter</u> :

- The diameter of a wire (d) corresponds to the diameter of its cross-sectional area. Tissue trauma is greater with larger gauge wires. Needle-set wires have a diameter close to that of the needle.

There are 2 nomenclatures for measuring the diameter of a wire:

- The USP standard (United State Pharmacopea): includes a notion of linear resistance for a given diameter. It is expressed in a certain number of 0's. Thus, the lower the resistance of the wire, the more there is to define it (7> 0 > 2/0 > 3/0...> 11/0).

The USP standard ranges from 7 to 11/0. Two yarns of the same diameter and different composition may have a different USP name. Two wires of the same diameter and different composition may have the same USP name.

- Decimal numbering: much simpler to use, it takes into account the diameter of the wire in 1/10th of a millimetre. Thus a wire with a decimal number of 2 will have a diameter of 0.2 mm. This numbering admits tolerances: Ex: dec 2 = 0,2 < Diameter <0,249 mm. The numbering

The decimal point ranges from O,l to 10.

<u>Equivalences between wire diameter and nomenclature</u> :

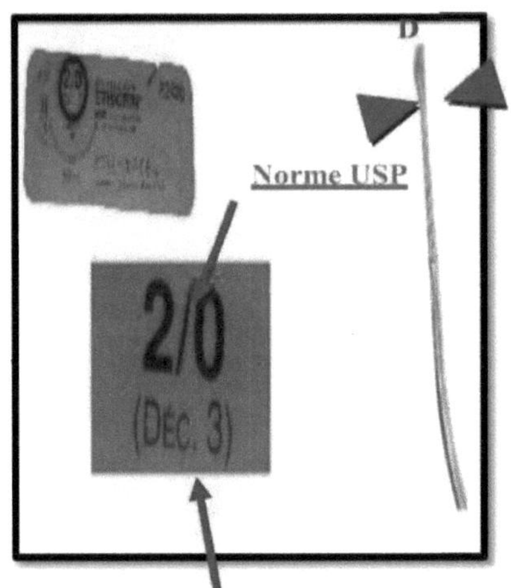

Decimal System
Figure: 03

Size in mm	Decimal system	USP' standard
0.02	0.2	10/0
0.03	0.3	9/0
0 .04	0.4	8/0
0.05	0.5	7/0
0.06	0.7	6/0
0.1	1	5/0
0.15	1.5	4/0
0.2	2	3/0
0.3	3	2/0
0.35	3.5	0
0.4	4	1
0.5	5	2
0.6	6	3.4
0.7	7	5
0.8	8	6
0.9	9	7

Table: 01

❖ <u>Tensile strength :</u>

- The tensile strength of a suture should be maximised in the immediate postoperative phase. To avoid disunion, the loss of strength of the wire over time must be balanced with the gain in strength of the surgical wound.

- Initially, the strength of the thread should be at least equal to the tensile strength of the fabric to be sutured.

- At the knot, the tensile strength of the yarn is halved.

❖ <u>Flexibility :</u>

- The flexibility of a wire is determined by its diameter and its nature. The larger the wire, the less flexible it is.

- Flexibility should be maintained or even increased in wet environments.

- Braided yarns are more manageable than monofilaments.

- Silk is the most flexible yarn.

❖ <u>Safety of the node:</u>

- The more slippery, stiff and heavy gauge the wire, the more likely the knot will come undone.

- Some yarns tend to return to their original shape after the knots have been tied, this is called yarn memory.

- The memory of a yarn is its ability to return to the shape it had when it came out of the package.

- A braided yarn has no memory in a wet environment.

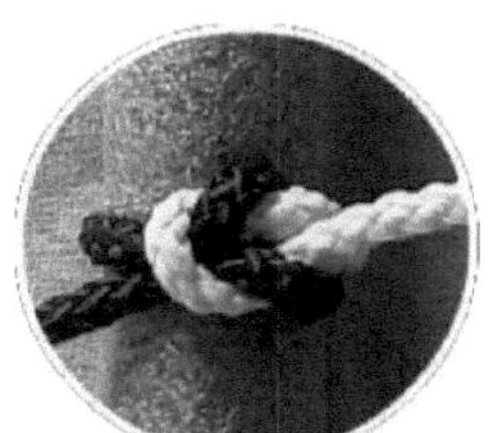

Figure: 04

❖ <u>Surface characteristics and coating :</u>

- Some braided threads are coated with a coating (Teflon, silicone, calcium stearate, etc.) which improves the gliding properties through the tissue and reduces the initial capillarity of the braid. The coated thread clings less, thus avoiding iatrogenic lesions caused by friction.

- Braided yarns are rougher than monofilaments.

    ❖ <u>Capillarity :</u>

- Characteristic in which fluids and bacteria remain attached and migrate along the thread.
- A braided yarn is a capillary yarn. The capillarity of a yarn is reduced when it is coated.
- Monofilaments are acapillary.

3.1.2 <u>Biological properties :</u>

    ❖ <u>Suturing and healing :</u>

- The suture is a foreign body that can prevent the normal healing process.
- Natural threads cause a more intense inflammatory reaction than synthetic threads.
- Too many stitches or too thick stitches prevent the healing process from running smoothly.

    ❖ <u>Suturing and infection:</u>

- Sutures, especially braided sutures (with gaps between the fibres), protect germs from phagocytosis (polyglycolic acid is said to release agents with antibacterial action).
- Absorbable monofilaments are preferred.

3.2 <u>Presentation:</u>

The yarns can be packaged in two forms:

- Needle-set (thread with a needle): Several types of packaging have been devised by manufacturers to improve thread extraction and reduce the memory effect (opposite).
- In reels (less expensive): useful for vascular ligations.

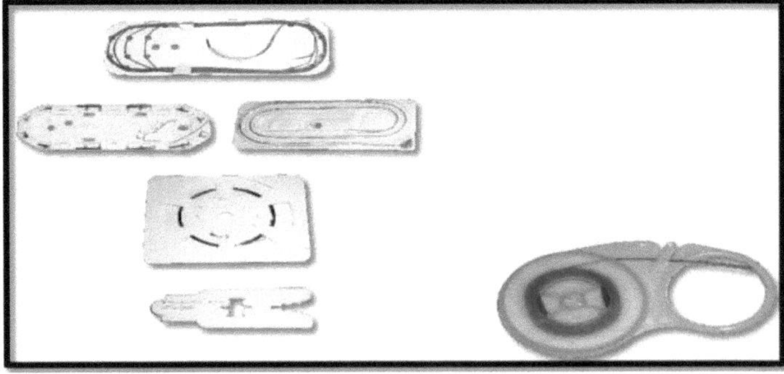

Figure: 05

3.3 <u>Needles :</u>

3.3.1 <u>Description :</u>

- The hands are made of stainless steel and consist of a point, a body and a heel.

- At the heel is the area where the thread is inserted into the needle.

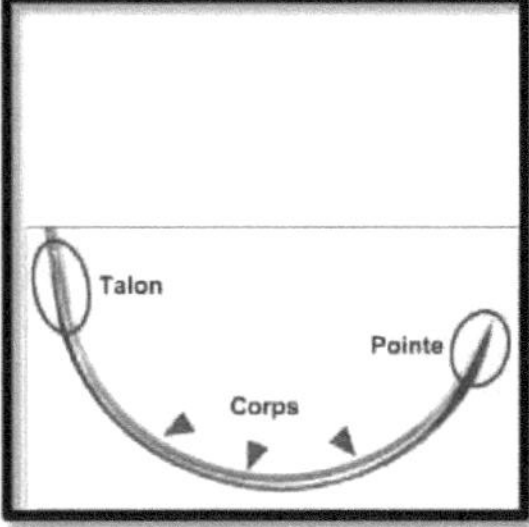

Figure: 06

❖ Heel:

- At present, almost all the threads used are crimped. The wire is inserted and then enclosed at the heel. These can be open channel (gutter) or hollow heel (drilled) needles. Crimping minimises the difference in diameter between the needle (d) and the wire (d'), thus reducing tissue trauma.
- Note: In small animal surgery, multi-use needles are no longer used because the difference in diameter between the wire (d) and the needle (d') is too great. Tissue trauma and septic risks are greater.

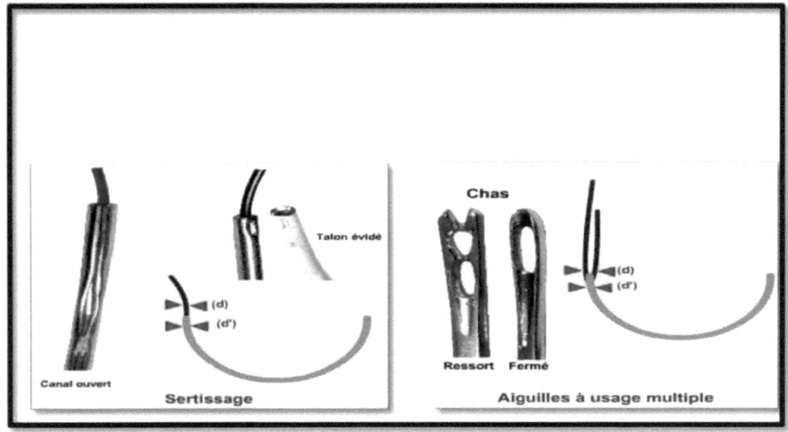

Figure: 07

3.3.2 Needle characteristics :

❖ Length (L):

- The length (L) of the needle is the distance from the tip to the heel. It should be sufficient to load both edges of a surgical wound in one go.

- The length of the needle can vary from 1-2 mm (for microsurgical needles) to over 70 mm.
- The typical length is between 20 and 30 mm.

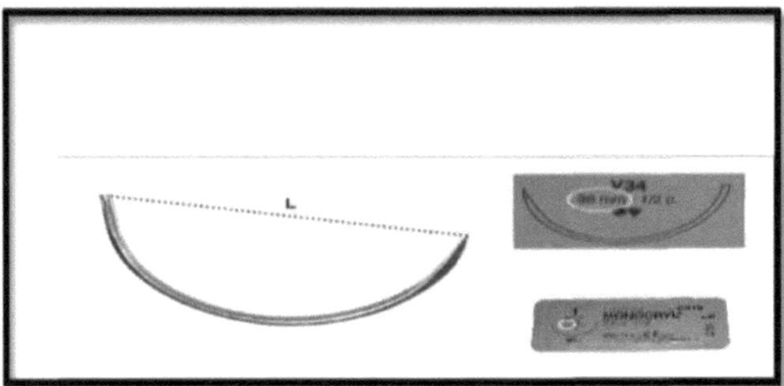

Figure: 08

❖ <u>Form:</u>

- Curvature
- The curvature of a needle is expressed in eighths of circles.
- The deeper the suture, the more eighths of a circle the curvature will need.

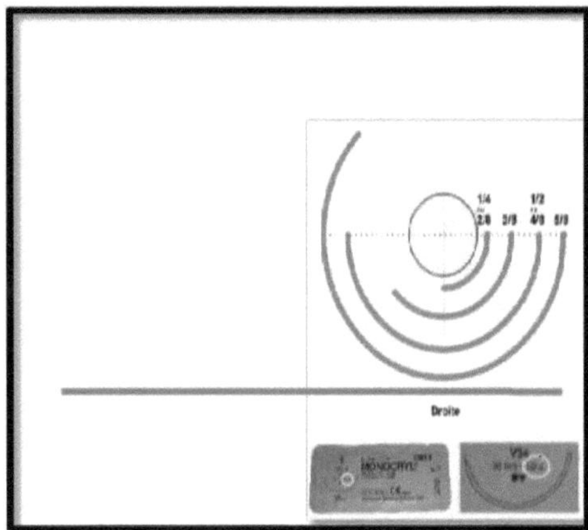

Figure: 09

Right	Suture of the superficial planes
1/4 circle	Used in ophthalmology, mainly.

3/8 circle	The most frequently used on superficial or wide planes.
1/2 circle	Used on small wounds, medium deep locations.
5/8 circle	Reserved for sutures of poorly accessible or deep wounds

Table: 02

❖ <u>Needle cross-section</u>:

The choice of the shape of the needle's cutting edge depends on the type of organ to be sutured. However, we can classify the needles into :

- Sharp needles

- Triangular or "Regular Cutting" needle. △ or ▲

Abandoned in favour of reverse cutting.

- Reverse triangle needle or "Reverse Cutting". ▽ or ▼

- The 3 sharp edges of the needle tip cut through the tissue, ensuring better penetration, especially in strong tissue.

- The edge formed by the apex of the triangle is directed downwards (on the concave side of the needle). The aim is to reduce the risk of tearing the tissue between the strands of the thread once the knot is tightened.

- The use of these needles is recommended on the skin, subcutaneous connective tissue, larynx, trachea, bronchi, external auditory canal, auricle, etc.

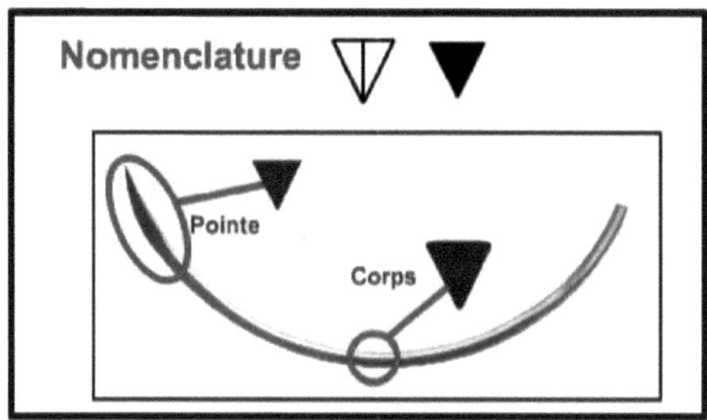

Figure: 10

- Spatula Point or Spatula Needle.

- These needles are used in ophthalmology.

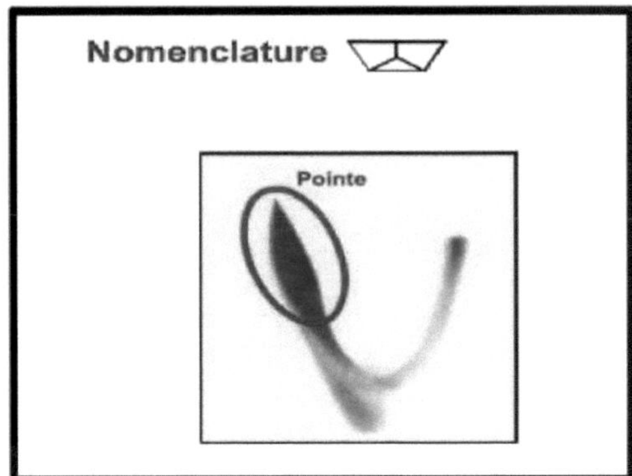

Figure: 11

❖ <u>Atraumatic needles:</u>

Pointeronde-Corpsarrondiou'TaperPoint'. 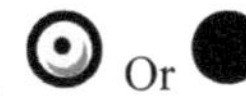 Or

-These needles pass through the organs, pulling apart the tissue as they go.

-Their use is reserved for digestive, urinary, vascular, subcutaneous sutures and in general for all sutures of fragile tissue.

VISIBLACK LASER®: Latest generation of round-tipped needles with a rounded body characterised by a better capacity for tissue penetration (less trauma).

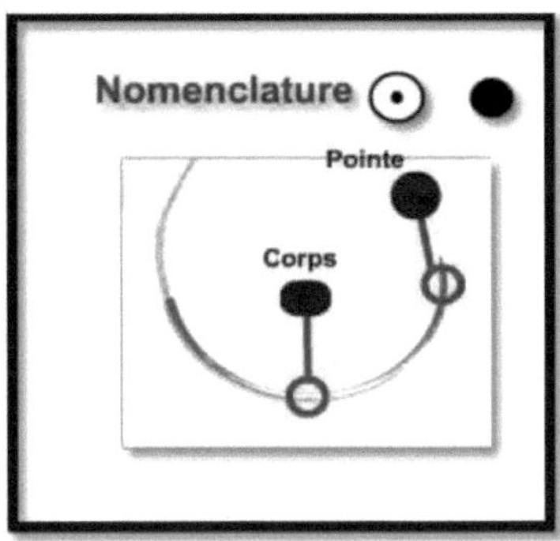

Figure: 12

- Blunt Point - Rounded body or "Blunt Point".

- These needles pass through the organs, pulling apart the tissue as they go.

- Their use is reserved for suturing friable organs (liver).

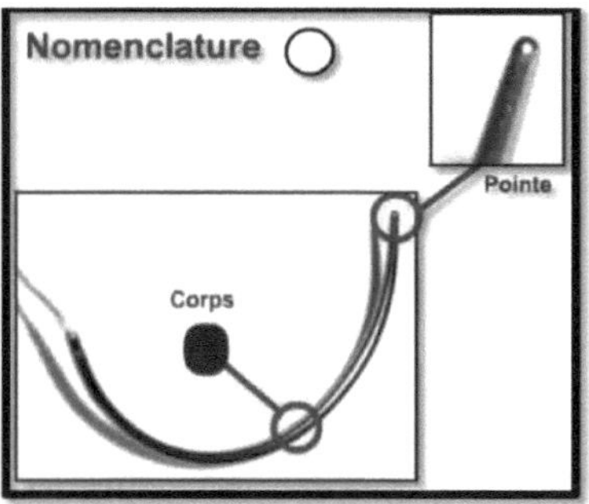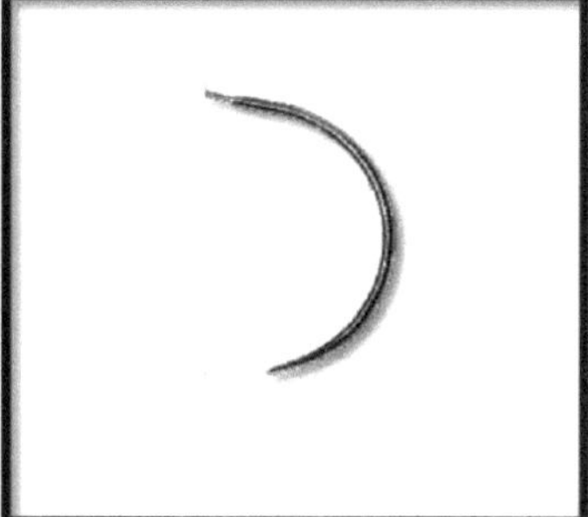

Figure : 13

❖ <u>Mixed needles:</u>

- Triangular tip - Rounded body or "Taper Cut". Or

These needles are triangular at the tip and rounded at the body:

- The triangular tip provides a penetration quality close to that of reverse cutting.

- The rounded body causes less tissue trauma when the needle is passed.

The use of this type of needle is recommended when suturing tendons, white line, trachea, tongue, nose, pads, fragile skin...

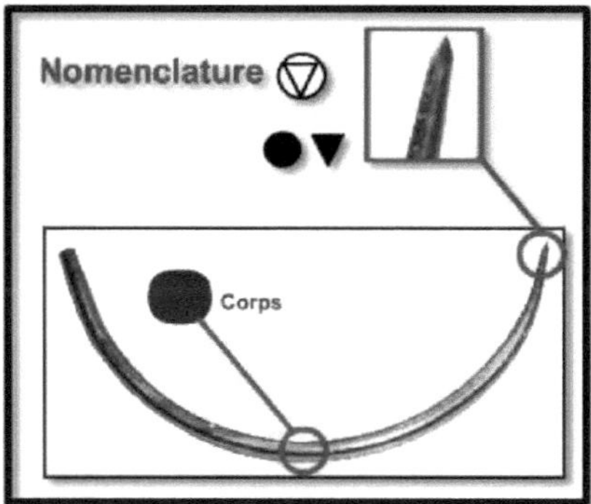

Figure: 14

❖ <u>Other needles :</u>

- Lancet needles. These needles are used in ophthalmology.

3.4 <u>Queue types :</u>

3.4.1 <u>Absorbable braids :</u>

❖ <u>Polyglycolic acid:</u>

Nature: polymer of glycolic acid.

Resistance time: 14 days.

Mode & time of total resorption: hydrolysis in 100-120 days.

Knot strength/security: good.

Tissue reaction: moderate at first and weak during resorption.

Tensile strength: average but decreasing rapidly.

Handling: average.

Dénominations commerciales : - Dexon S® -Ercedex®

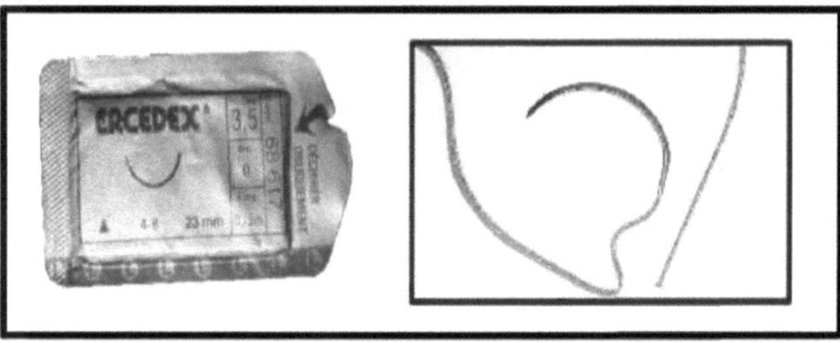

Figure: 15

This braided yarn tends to: return to the shape it had in its ballooning.

This "memory" tends to disappear in a humid environment.

❖ <u>Coated Polyglycolic Acid(Resorbable):</u>

Nature: Glycolic acid polymer coated with surfactant.

Resistance time: 14 days.

Mode & time of total resorption: hydrolysis in 100-120 days.

Knot strength/security: medium.

Tissue reaction: moderate at first and weak during resorption.

Tensile strength: medium and decreasing rapidly.

Handling: very good.

Trade names :

- The Dexon™

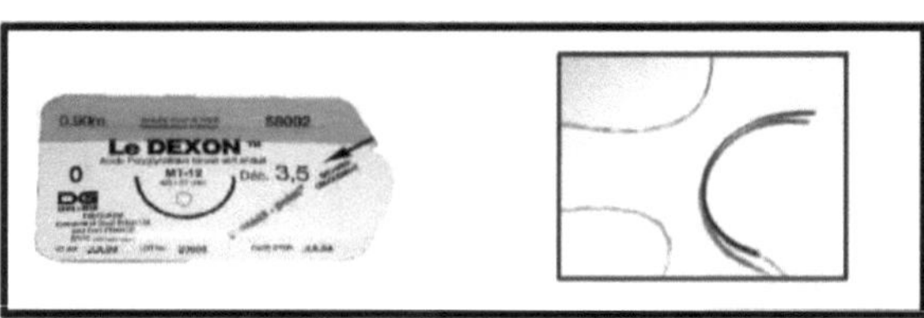

Figure : 14

This braided and coated yarn takes on the shape it had in its packaging. This memory disappears in a humid environment.

❖ LACTOMER*(Resorbable)

Nature: Glycolide/lactide copolymer (derived from glycolic acid and lactic acid) coated with a mixture of caprolactone/glycolide copolymer and calcium stearoyl lactylate.

Resistance time: 25-28 days.

Mode & time of total resorption: hydrolysis in 60-70 days.

Knot strength / security: medium.

Tissue reaction: weak.

Tensile strength: medium.

Handling: good.

Trade names: - POLYSORB

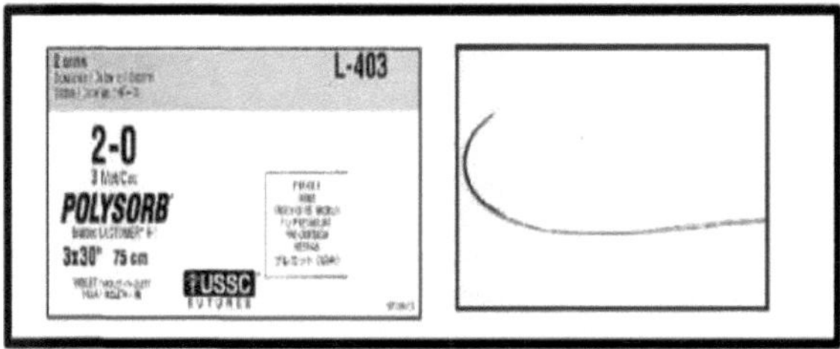

Figure: 17

The memory of this yarn disappears in a wet environment.

❖ Polyglactin 910 irradiated: (Resorbable)

Nature: Copolymer of glycolic acid and lactic acid coated with calcium stearate and sterilised by irradiation.

Resistance time: 10-12 days.

Mode & time of total resorption: hydrolysis in 42 days.

Knot strength/security: good.

Tissue reaction: weak.

Tensile strength: medium.

Handling: average.

Trade names: - VICRYL ® fast.

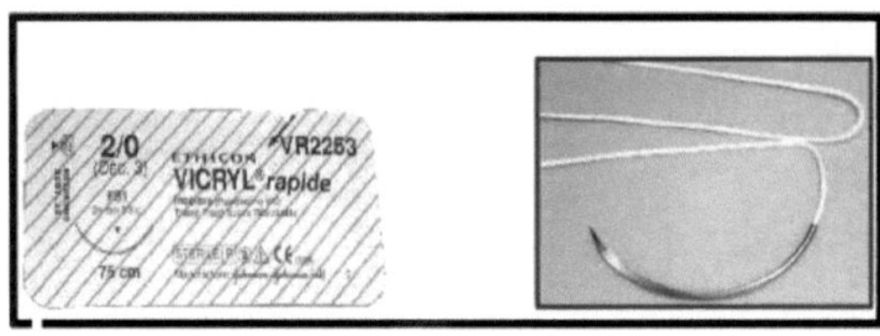

Figure: 18

The memory of this yarn disappears in a wet environment.

❖ <u>Polyglactin 910</u> :(Resorbable)

Nature: Copolymer of acid and lactic acid coated with calcium stearate.

Resistance time: 28 days.

Mode & time of total resorption: hydrolysis in 56-70 days.

Knot strength/security: good.

Tissue reaction: weak.

Tensile strength: good.

Handling: average.

Trade names: - VICRYL ®

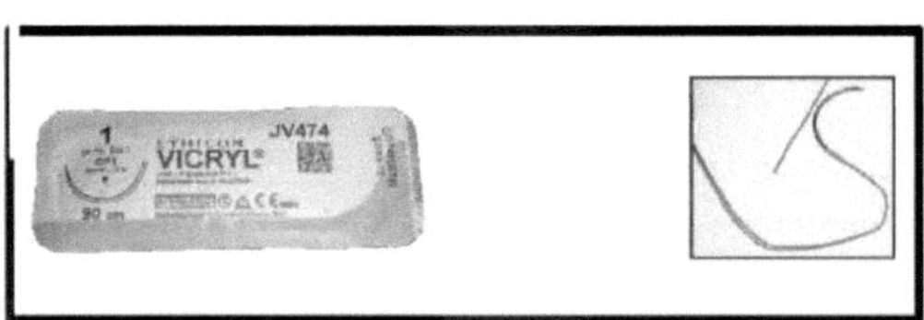

Figure: 19

This braided and coated yarn tends to return to the shape it had in its packaging. This memory disappears in a humid environment.

3.4.2   <u>Absorbable monobrins :</u>

❖ <u>GLYCOMER* 631:</u> (Absorbable monofilament)

Nature: glycolide (60%), dioxanone (14%) and trimethylene carbonate (26%).

Resistance time: 30 days.

Mode & time of total resorption: hydrolysis in 90-110 days.

Knot strength/security: good.

Tissue reaction: weak.

Tensile strength: intermediate.

Handling: very good.

Trade names: - BIOSYN

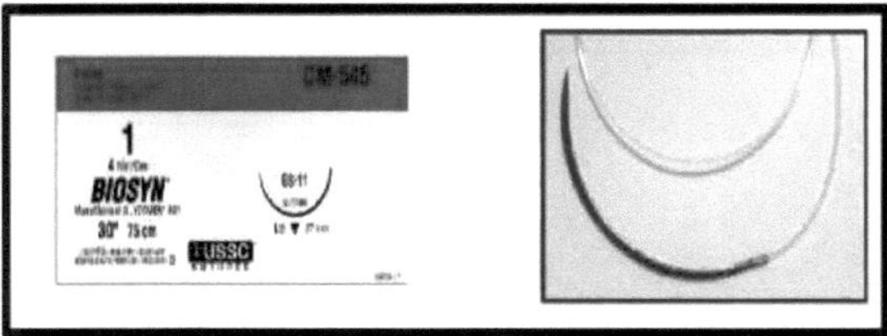

Figure: 20

This monofilament has little memory.

❖ <u>Poliglecaprone 25: (Absorbable monofilament)</u>

Nature: copolymer of glycolic acid and trimethylene carbonate.

Resistance time: 15-20 days.

Mode & time of total resorption: hydrolysis in 90-120 days.

Knot strength/security: good.

Tissue reaction: moderate at first and weak during resorption. Tensile strength: strong initially (the best of the resorbable monofilaments) then decreases rapidly.

Handling: excellent.

Trade names: - MONOCRYL® (a), (b), (c), (d), (e), (f) and (g)

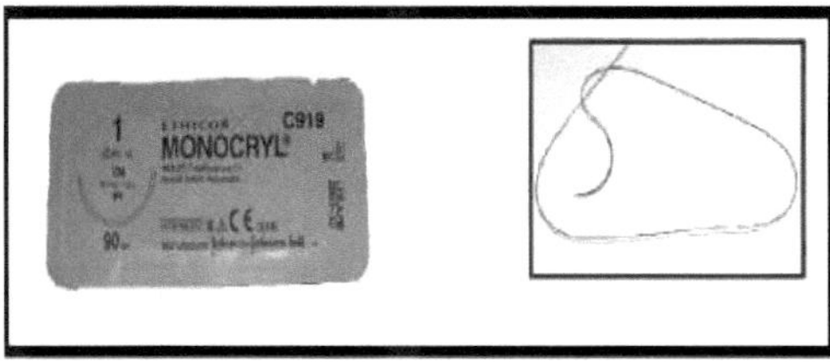

Figure: 21

This monofilament tends to return to the shape it had in its packaging.

❖ <u>Polydioxanone;(Resorbable monofilament)</u>

Nature: Polymer of paradioxanone.

Resistance time: 55 days.

Mode & time of total resorption: hydrolysis in 180-210 days.

Knot strength/security: good.

Tissue reaction: moderate at first and weak during resorption.

Tensile strength: good.

Handling: very good.

Trade names: - PDS® II

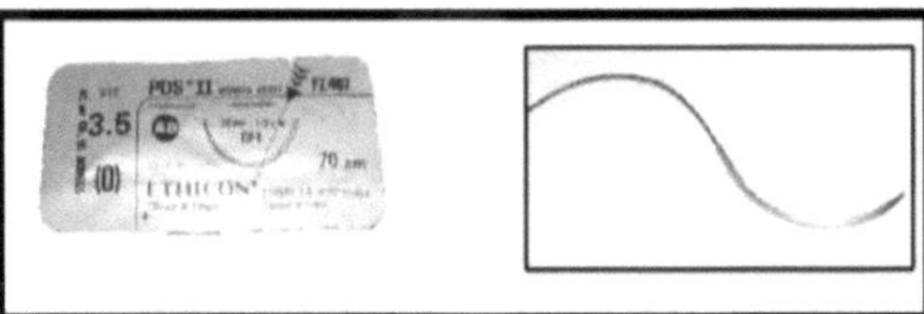

Figure: 22

This monofilament has little memory.

❖ Polyglyconate:(Absorbable monofilament)

Nature: copolymer of glycolic acid and trimethylene carbonate.

Resistance time: 30 days.

Mode & time of total resorption: hydrolysis in 180 days.

Knot strength/security: good.

Tissue reaction: moderate at first and weak during resorption.

Tensile strength: good.

Handling: very good.

Trade names: - MAXON*

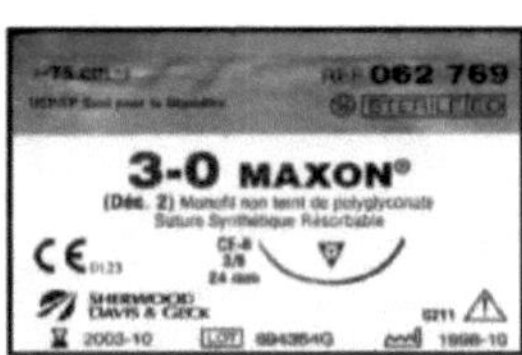

Figure: 23

3.4.3 Non-resorbable braids :

❖ Braided polyester: (Irresorbable)

Nature: synthetic resin polymer.

Resistance time: non-absorbable, and excellent resistance retention.

Knot strength/security: poor.

Tissue reaction: quite strong.

Tensile strength: high.

Handling: good.

Trade names: - MERSUTURES - SURGIDAC*.

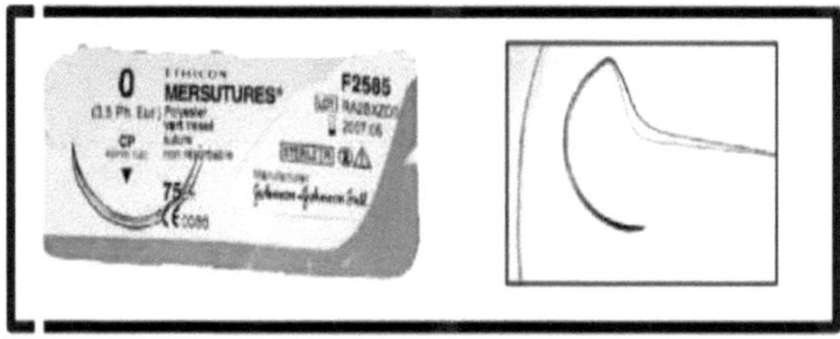

Figure: 24

This thread has very little memory.

❖ <u>Coated braided polyester: (Irresorbable)</u>

Nature: synthetic resin polymer coated with Teflon or silicone.

Resistance time: the coating breaks down over time and increases the reaction of the tissue.

Knot strength/security: average to poor.

Tissue reaction: quite strong.

Tensile strength: high.

Handling: good.

Trade names: - ETHIBOND - LIGALENE - ERCYLENE

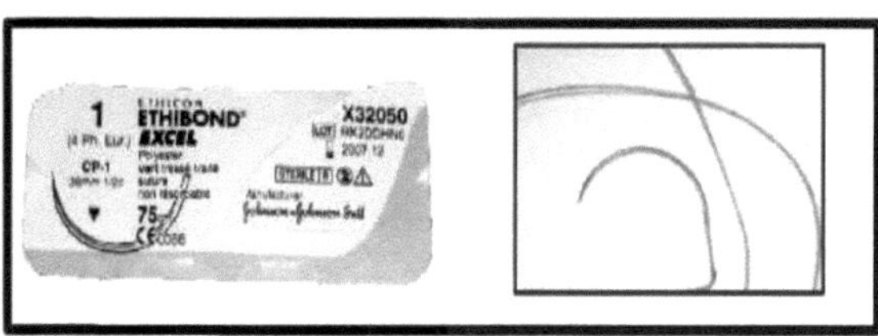

Figure: 25

This thread has a low memory.

❖ <u>Braided silk:</u>

Nature: silkworm thread Resistance time: 30% loss of initial resistance at 14 days and 50% at 1 year.

Knot strength/security: good.

Tissue reaction: significant.

Tensile strength: medium.

Handling: excellent.

Trade names: - SILK - SOFSILK®.

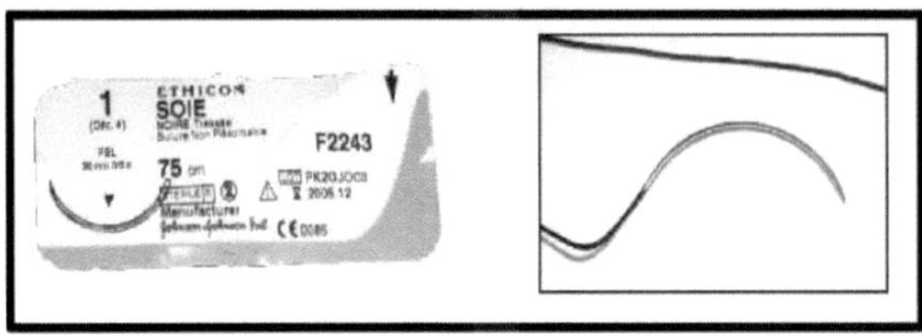

Figure: 26

This thread has little memory.

3.4.4 Non-resorbable monobrins :

❖ Nylon: (Irresorbable monofilament)

Nature: polyamide.

Resistance time: resistance decreases by 10-20% per year.

Knot strength/security: average (poor for large sizes).

Tissue reaction: weak.

Tensile strength: intermediate.

Handling: average to poor.

Trade names: - ETHILON® - ETHICRIN® - CRINERCE*

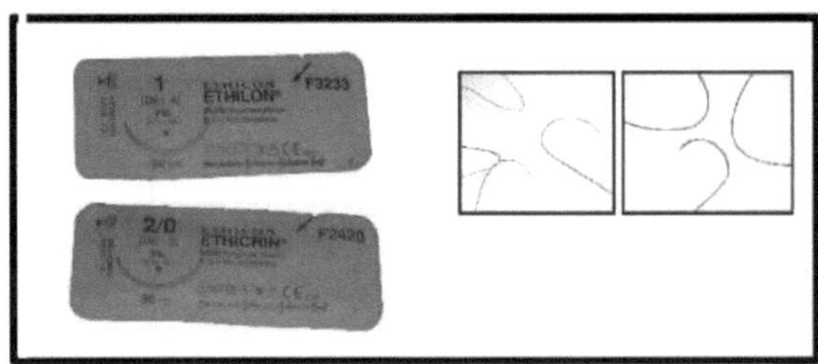

Figure: 27

Note the difference in memory between these two threads.

Packaged, ETHILON® is immersed in an alcohol solution.

❖ Polypropylene: (Irresorbable monofilament)

Nature: hydrocarbon polymer.

Resistance time: no change in resistance over time.

Knot strength/security: excellent (average for large sizes).

Tissue reaction: very weak.

Tensile strength: very good.

Handling: good to average.

Trade names: - PROLENE® - SURGIPRO*

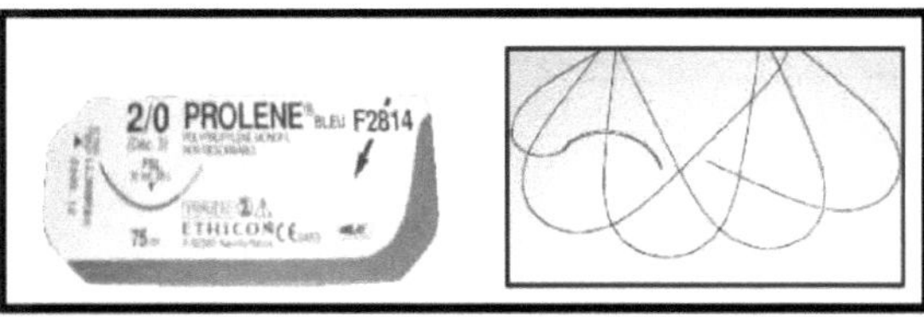

Figure: 28

The yarn tends to return to the shape it had in its packaging.

3.4.5 Metal monoblock :

❖ Steel: (Irresorbable monofilament)

Type: stainless steel.

Resistance time: poor resistance to bending.

Knot strength/security: excellent.

Tissue reaction: very weak. The heads of the knots can create inflammation or even necrosis

by friction. Tensile strength: high.

Handling: average.

Trade names: - STEEL

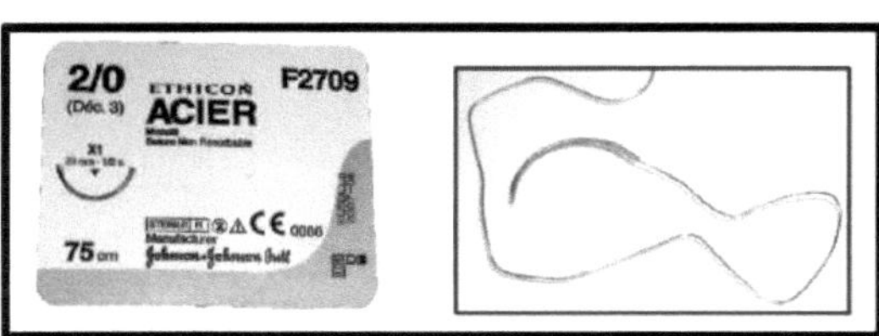

Figure 29: This wire has no "memory".

CHAPTER 2

<u>Suture technique:</u>

- Basic elements.

- Main entanglements.

- Separate points.

- Overspray.

<u>II / Suturing technique :</u>

1. <u>Basic elements :</u>

1.1 <u>Single half node :</u>

- Technical :

- The cheflong is wrapped around the needle holder held between the two strands.

- The short leader is gripped between the jaws and then tied to the long leader by crossing it symmetrically in relation to the median axis.

- Tightening is done by pulling the two strands symmetrically in opposite directions. It is essential that the two strands are in line with each other.

- Note:

- In order to limit the effects of traction on the pedicle or tissue, it is important that the tensile forces on both strands are equal.

- Due to the crossing, the short leader that was originally on one side is on the opposite side after the half knot is executed.

1.2   <u>Reverse half node :</u>

-Technical :

- The cheflong is wrapped around the needle holder held on the outside.

- The short leader is gripped between the jaws and then tied to the long leader by crossing it symmetrically in relation to the median axis.

- Tightening is done by pulling the two strands symmetrically in opposite directions. It is essential that the two strands are in line with each other.

- Note:

- In order to limit the effects of traction on the pedicle or tissue, it is important that the tensile forces exerted on the two strands are equal.

- Due to the crossing, the short leader that was originally on one side is on the opposite side after the half knot is executed.

1.3 Transforming a half node into a key :

- Technical :
- The half knot is loosened beforehand.
- The short leader is seized and stretched towards oneself.
- The cheflong is placed on the opposite side.
- Clamping is done by sliding the cheflong towards the surgical site.
- Note:
- As a half-key is made without crossing the strands, it is important to remember to uncross the strands when processing.
- The two strands must form a right angle during tightening.

1.4 Half of the chi ru rgi en :

-Technical :
- The long leader is wound two turns on the needle holder held between the two strands.
- The short leader is gripped between the bits and then tied to the long leader by crossing the latter symmetrically in relation to the median axis.
- Tightening is done by pulling the two strands symmetrically in opposite directions. It is essential that the two strands are in line with each other.
-Note:
- In order to limit the effects of traction on the pedicle or tissue, it is important that the tensile forces on both strands are equal.
- Due to the crossing, the short leader that was originally on one side is on the opposite side after the half knot is executed.

1.5 Half-key "short leader" :

-Technical :
- The cheflong is wrapped around the needle holder held between the two strands.
- The short leader is gripped between the jaws and stretched towards oneself.

- The clamping is done by sliding the long head over the short head in the direction of the Operating Field.

- Remarks :

- When tightening, the two strands form a right angle and the short head should be kept taut towards you.

- In contrast to the half knot, the short leader which was initially on one side is on the same side after the half knot has been executed.

1.6 Half key "long leader" :

-Technical :

- The cheflong is wrapped around the needle holder held between the two strands.

- The cheflong is stretched towards you.

- The clamping is done by sliding the short head over the long head in the direction of the surgical site.

- Remarks :

- When tightening, the two strands form a right angle and the long head should be kept taut towards you.

- In contrast to the half knot, the short leader which was initially on one side is on the same side after the half knot has been executed.

1.7 Transformation of a half-key into a half-node d :

- Technical :

- The half-key is loosened beforehand.

- The short leader is seized and stretched towards oneself.

- The cheflong is transposed to the opposite side.

- The short leader is aligned in line with the long leader.

- Tightening is done by pulling the two strands symmetrically in opposite directions.

- Note:

- As a half knot is made by crossing the strands, you must not forget to cross the strands when processing.

- When tightening, it is essential that the two strands are in line with each other.

1.6   Double half key "cheflong":

- Technical :

- Execution of a "cheflong" half key.

- Tightening the half-key.

- Execution of the second "cheflong" half-key.

- Tighten the second half-key.

- Note:

- These two half-keys slide on the same head (long) and can thus perfect the tightening once the second one is in place.

1.7   half key achieved :

- Technical :

Interesting for vascular ligations, wall approximation, tightening of osteo-articular prostheses...

-A double half-key is not considered a knot and is called a "false knot" or "slip knot" and must be completed (see Complete keys).

1.8   Double half-key "chef court":

- Technical :

- Execution of a "short leader" half key.

- Tightening the half-key.

- Execution of the second half key "short leader".

- Tighten the second half-key.

- Note:

- These two half-keys can slide over the short head and thus complete the tightening once the second one is in place.

2. Main entanglements :

2.1   Complete keys (long head or short head) :

- Technical :

- Making a double "cheflong" or "chef court" half-key.

- Tighten by sliding the two half keys onto one of the strands.

- Execute and tighten a third half-key in the opposite direction to the first two.

- A fourth half-key can be added in the same direction as the first two.

- Note:

- In this type of interlocking, the tightening of the second half-key allows the carrying wire of these half-keys to slide and thus allows a possible re-tightening.

- The execution of the third half-key in the opposite direction ensures the blocking of the enclosure achieved by the first two half-keys.

- This is used for vascular ligations, for tightening certain ligament prostheses or for bringing together tissues under great tension.

2.2 <u>Single or double reverse half key</u>:

-Technical :

- Execution of a half key.

- Tightening the half-key.

- Execute a second half-key in the opposite direction to the first.

- Tighten the second half-key.

-Note:

The single key does not loosen once the second half key is tightened.

2.3 <u>"Cow knot" or asymmetric knot</u>:

- Technical :

This node consists of two half nodes:

- Undemi-knot made   with the needle holder between the strands.

- A half inverted knot made with the needle holder worn.

Externally on the side of the long head.

- Note:

- Bad knot: loosens easily after tightening.

- By pulling on the wire loops near the binding, the knot moves back and loosens.

2.4 <u>"Pl at knot" or "straight knot" or symmetrical knot</u>:

- Technical :

This knot consists of similar half knots.

- Note:

- Good knot, does not loosen after tightening.

- By pulling on the wire loops near the binding, the knot does not recede and is tightened.

   3.   <u>Separate points:</u>

   3.4 <u>Single point:</u>

- Technical :

- The needle passes through the first bank from the outside to the inside and then through the second bank from the inside to the outside.

- The chiefs are then knotted and tightened next to the line formed by the wound.

- Note:

- When tightening, the wire penetration points tend to come into contact, causing the edges to turn towards the side where the knot is located, especially if they are stretched before being tied.

- To prevent the banks from turning over, the wire should be knotted before it is tensioned.

- Advantage:

In case of infection, the stitches can be removed without destroying the entire suture.

   3.5 <u>Reverse single stitch or concealed knot</u> :

- Technical :

- The needle passes through the first bank from the inside to the outside and through the second bank from the outside to the inside.

- The leaders are then tied and tightened. The knot is then buried under the banks.

- Note:

- When tightening, the wire penetration points tend to come into contact, causing the edges to turn towards the side where the knot is located.

- The burial of the knot forces the surgeon to use an absorbable suture.

- Used in all cases where there is no risk of high tensions.

- Advantage:

- Reduces discomfort or chafing caused by the suture knot.

- Buried nodes are inaccessible.

   3.6 <u>Single point in the slice</u> :

- Technical :

- The needle penetrates the first bank to emerge in the thickness of the dermis. On the second bank, the needle is introduced into the thickness of the dermis to emerge at the surface.

- The leaders are then tied and tightened.

- Note:

- At the moment of tightening, the wire penetration points will come into contact, causing the two edges to clash.

- Thin tissue cannot be sutured with this type of suture.

- Used in all cases where there is no risk of high tensions.

-Advantage:

Face the banks.

3.7 Reverse single stitch in the edge :

- Technical :

- From the inside out, the needle passes through the subcutaneous connective tissue to emerge in the thickness of the dermis of the first bank.

- From the outside in, the needle is inserted into the thickness of the dermis of the second bank and passes through it and the subcutaneous connective tissue.

- The leaders are then tied and tightened.

- Note:

- At the moment of tightening, the wire penetration points will come into contact, causing the two edges to clash.

- The burial of the knot forces the surgeon to use an absorbable suture.

- Thin tissue cannot be sutured with this type of suture.

- Used in all cases where there is no risk of high tensions.

- Advantage:

- Face the banks.

- Reduces discomfort or chafing caused by knots.

- Buried nodes are inaccessible.

3.8 Reversing U-point:

- Technical :

- The needle goes through the first bank from the outside to the inside and then, further on the same bank, it is pricked from the inside to the outside

- The same principle is applied to the second bank.

- The leaders are tied and then tightened.
- Remarks :
- When tightened, the edges tend to turn inwards, especially if they are stretched and crossed before being knotted.
- To prevent the banks from turning over, the wire should be knotted before it is tensioned.
- Advantage:
- U-stitches allow the edges of a wound to be joined together quickly and securely.
- This suturing technique reverses the edges of a wound.

3.9 Splayed U-point:

- Technical :
- The needle passes through the first bank from the outside to the inside and then through the second bank from the inside to the outside.
- Further on, on the latter, the first bank is pricked from the outside to the inside and finally from the inside to the outside.
- The leaders are tied and then tightened.
- Note:
- When tightening, the edges tend to turn outwards, especially if the leaders are stretched and crossed before being knotted.
- To prevent the banks from turning over, the wire should be knotted before it is tensioned.
- Advantage:
- The U-stitches allow the edges of a wound to be joined together quickly and securely.
- This suturing technique allows for eversion of the wound edges.

3.10 X-point :

- Technical :
- The needle passes through the first bank from the outside to the inside and then perpendicularly from the inside to the outside of the second bank.
- The needle passes obliquely inwards through the first bank and then perpendicularly through the second bank from the inside to the surface.
- The chiefs are then knotted and tightened next to the line formed by the wound.
- Note:
- The crossing of the X-wires is done on the outside.

- A variant is to obtain the X-crossing on the inside.
- Advantage:

The X point faces the banks.

3.11 <u>Point de Lembert :</u>

- Technical :
- The spike is placed between 0.5 and 1 cm from the edge of the first bank.

The needle passes through the adventitia and muscularis to exit at the edge of the wound (on the same bank).

- On the second bank, the stitches are made in the same way as above, close to the edge of the wound, to emerge on the surface 0.5-1 cm from the edge, still perpendicular to the line of incision.
- The leaders are then tied and tightened.
- Note:
- At no time should the mucosa be crossed.
- This type of suture is used for hollow organs requiring reversal of the edges.
- Advantage:
- Reverses wound edges
- The tensile forces are distributed over 4 points.

3.12 <u>Modified Lembert Point:</u>

- Technical :
- The needle is inserted between 0.5 and 1 cm from the edge of the first bank, passing through the serosal and muscular layers to the submucosa and out onto the surface of the same bank, close to and perpendicular to the edge.
- On the second bank, the stitches are made in the same way as above, close to the edge of the wound, to emerge 0.5-1 cm further back, parallel to the line of incision.
- The pin is inserted near the edge of the first bank, perpendicularly, to emerge 0.5-1 cm further out, at the surface.
- The leaders are then tied and tightened.
- Note:
- At no time should the mucosa be crossed.

- This type of suture is used for hollow organs requiring reversal of the edges.
- Advantage:
- Reverses the wound edges.
- The tensile forces are distributed over 6 points.

3.13   Gambee point :

- Technical :
- The needle is inserted close to the edge of the first bank, which is crossed from side to side. On this same bank, the needle is passed through the mucosa and submucosa without reaching the muscularis.

The needle comes out in the slice, without reaching the surface.

- The second bank is approached from the edge, passing inwards through the submucosal and mucosal layers and then exiting outwards, close to the edge of the wound, passing through all the layers including the serosa.
- The leaders are then tied and tightened.
- Note:
- This suture faces the banks edge to edge.
- This type of suture is used for intestinal anastomoses.
- Advantage:

Face the edges of the wound.

3.11   No "far-from-near-far":

- Technical :
- You prick, from the outside in, 0.5-1 cm from the edge of the first bank (far).
- In the opposite direction, you cross the second bank close to the edge (close).
- The first bank is crossed close to the edge, from the outside to the inside (close).
- In the opposite direction, 0.5-1 cm from the edge of the second bank, the needle came to the surface (far).
- The leaders are then tied and tightened.
- Note:

The "far" and "near" components may be slightly offset.

- Advantage:
- Face the edges of the wound.

- The tensile forces are distributed over 4 points.

- Useful when the edges of a wound are weakened.

3.12 Halsted point :

- Technical :

- Making a Lembert stitch.

- Parallel to the wound edge, at a distance of 0.5-1 cm, a second Lembert stitch is made in the opposite direction.

- The leaders are then tied and tightened.

- Note:

- At no time should the mucosa be crossed.

- This type of suture is used for hollow organs requiring reversal of the edges.

- Advantages:

- Reverses the wound edges.

- The tensile forces are distributed over 8 points.

- Useful on weakened organs.

4. Overlays :

4.1 Start of overlocking :

- Technical :

- A simple stitch is made (the U-stitch is also valid in case of fragile fabrics). The short head is cut and the long head is preserved.

- In the case of Lembert overlock, the first stitch is a simple Lembert.

- The single stitch used to start a Cushing's overlay should not cross the entire thickness of the edges.

4.2 End of overlock :

- Technical :

An overlay is completed by making a knot with the leaders on either side of the surgical wound:

- First head: crimped strand.

- Second chief: consisting of the last loose loop of the overlock.

The strands are knotted and then tightened.

4.3   <u>Simple overlock</u> :

- Technical :

- Making a simple stitch while preserving the crimped cheflong.

- The first bank is crossed, then perpendicular to the line of incision, the second bank is crossed.

- On the first bank, 0.5-1 cm from the first penetration point, the above step is repeated along the wound.

- The handles are tightened at each needle exit.

- On the last point, the last loop is not tightened, it will be tied with the end of the thread.

- Note:

- The visible loops are oblique, the buried wire is perpendicular to the incision line.

- A variant of this overlay is to obtain visible loops perpendicular to the incision line.

- Each time the needle is passed, the edges of the incision must be faced.

- Clamping is carried out in such a way that there are no bulges or folds.

- Advantage:

- Tackle the edges

- Quick implementation

4.4   <u>Overlocking in "passé" or Reverdin stitch:</u>

- Technical :

The technique is identical to the simple overlocking technique with the only difference being that each time the second bank comes out, the thread is passed through the loop formed by the last loose loop.

- Note:

- The visible and hidden parts of the wire are perpendicular to the incision line.

- Each time the needle is passed, the edges of the incision must be faced.

- The clamping is done in such a way that there are no beads or folds.

- Advantage:

- The perpendicularity of the handles ensures that the edges are better aligned.

- Fast execution.

4.5   <u>Simple intradermal suture:</u>

- Technical :

- The first stitch is simple reversed, in the edge. The crimped cheflong is preserved.

- From the inside out, the needle passes through the subcutaneous connective tissue to emerge in the thickness of the dermis of the first bank.

- From the outside in, the needle is inserted into the thickness of the dermis of the second bank and passes through it and the subcutaneous connective tissue.

- This process is repeated along the surgical wound.

- The handles are tightened at each needle exit.

- On the last point, the last loop is not tightened, it will be tied with the end of the thread.

- Note:

- At the moment of tightening, the wire penetration points will come into contact, causing the two edges to clash.

- The burial of the knot forces the surgeon to use an absorbable suture.

- Thin tissue cannot be sutured with this type of suture.

- Used in all cases where there is no risk of high tensions.

- Advantage:

- Face the edges.

- Buried nodes are inaccessible.

- Fast execution.

4.6 <u>U-shaped intradermal suture:</u>

- Technical :

- The first stitch is simple reversed, in the edge. The long head is preserved.

- Parallel to the edge of the wound, the wound is punctured into the dermis and exited 0.5-1 cm further on.

- Opposite the last point of penetration, on the second bank, the same point is made and so along the incision line.

- The handles are tightened at each needle exit.

- On the last point, the last loop is not tightened, it will be tied with the end of the thread.

- Note:

- At the moment of tightening, the wire penetration points will come into contact, causing the two edges to clash.

- The burial of the knot forces the surgeon to use an absorbable suture.

- Thin tissue cannot be sutured with this type of suture.

- Used in all cases where there is no risk of high tensions.
- Advantage:
- Face the edges.
- Buried nodes are inaccessible.
- Fast execution.

4.7 Reverse U-joint:

- Technical :
- The first stitch is simple or U-shaped. The crimped cheflong is preserved.
- The first bank is pricked and then parallel to the incision line, at 0.5-1 cm, the same bank is crossed from the inside to the outside.
- The second bank is pricked perpendicular to the line of incision, from the outside inwards, and then 0.5-1 cm from the surface.
- The same process is repeated along the surgical wound.
- The handles are tightened at each needle exit.
- On the last point, the last loop is not tightened, it will be tied with the end of the thread.
- Note:
- When tightened, the banks tend to turn inwards.
- To prevent the edges from turning over, the thread should be slightly taut at each needle exit.
- Advantage:
- Reverses the wound edges.
- Fast execution.

4.8 U-shaped flaring or "quilting" overlock:

- Technical :
- The first stitch is simple or U-shaped. The crimped cheflong is preserved.
- The first bank is pricked, then the second bank is crossed perpendicular to the line of incision.
- The latter is re-crossed, 0.5-1 cm from the last point of exit of the wire.
- Perpendicular to the incision line, the first bank is pricked.
- The same process is repeated along the surgical wound.

- The handles are tightened at each needle exit.

- On the last point, the last loop is not tightened, it will be tied with the end of the thread.

- Note:

- When tightened, the banks tend to turn outwards.

- To prevent the edges from turning over, the thread should be slightly taut at each needle exit.

- Advantage:

- Everse the wound edges.

- Fast execution.

4.9 Lembert's overjet :

- Technical :

- The first point is simple in the slice or Lembert. The long crimped head is preserved.

- The first Lembert point is achieved.

- We return to the first bank to perform a second Lembert stitch.

- The suture is continued along the entire length of the surgical wound.

- The handles are tightened at each needle exit.

- On the last point, the last loop is not tightened, it will be tied with the end of the thread.

Note:

- At no time should the mucosa be crossed.

- This type of suture is used for hollow organs requiring reversal of the edges.

- Advantage:

- Reverses the wound edges.

- The tensile forces are distributed over 4 points.

4.9 Cushing's Surgery:

- Technical :

- The first stitch is simple in the edge. The crimped cheflong is preserved.

- Without crossing the mucosa, the needle is inserted and then withdrawn 0.5-1 cm, on the same bank and parallel to the incision line.

- Opposite the last point of penetration, the same operation is carried out on the second bank and all along the incision.

- The handles are tightened at each needle exit.
- On the last point, the last loop is not tightened, it will be tied with the end of the thread.
- Note:
- At no time should the mucosa be crossed.
- This type of suture is used for hollow organs requiring reversal of the edges.
- Advantage:
- Reverses the wound edges.

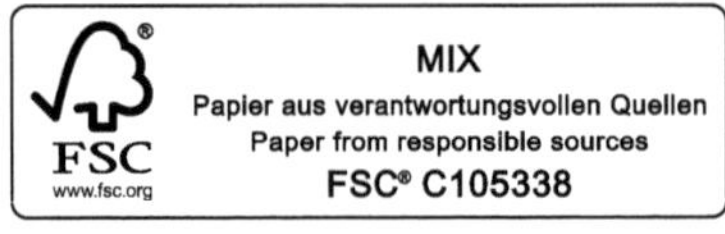

Printed by Books on Demand GmbH, Norderstedt / Germany